Building Great Relationships

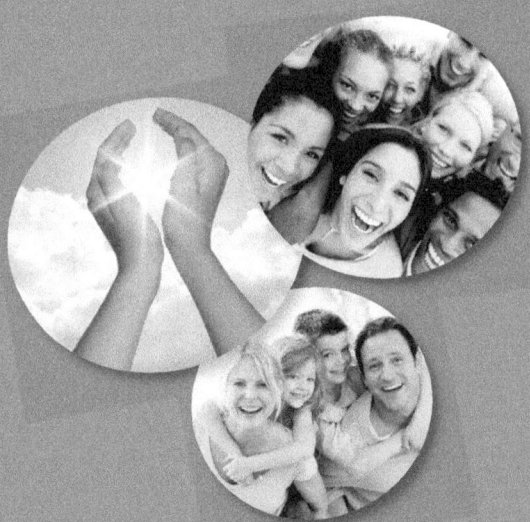

Building Great Relationships

by John Christopher

Contents

Building lasting and rewarding relationships

The best things in life – success, happiness, love – depend on your ability to create and maintain great relationships. Everyone puts their best foot forward in a new work setting or when looking to attract a mate, but often have problems trying to maintain their relationships over the long term. That's because keeping a relationship healthy and fulfilling, requires a set of emotional intelligence skills that many of us don't have.

These five emotional intelligence skills that are of vital importance in building and maintaining healthy relationships are:

Skill One: The ability to manage stress

Skill Two: The ability to recognize and manage your emotions

Skill Three: The ability to communicate nonverbally

Skill Four: The ability to use humour and play

Skill Five: The ability to resolve conflicts

Skill One - The ability to manage stress

The first skill for building rewarding and lasting relationships is the ability to manage stress. Stress shuts down your ability to feel, to think rationally, and to be emotionally available to another person, essentially blocking good communication. This damages the relationship. Being able to regulate stress allows you to remain emotionally available. The first step in communicating with emotional intelligence is recognizing when stress levels are out of control and returning yourself and others, whenever possible, to a relaxed and energized state of awareness.

You can face strong and even frightening emotions with comfort when you know how to manage stress. When you're under high levels of stress, rational thinking and decision making go out the window. Extreme stress overwhelms the mind and body, getting in the way of your ability to accurately read a situation. It makes it difficult to hear what someone else is saying, to be aware of your own feelings and needs, and prevents you from communicating clearly.

Learning how to quickly relieve stress and stay calm and focused in the moment will enable you to tackle challenges with a clear head. You will communicate clearly and powerfully even in tense situations. You will stay balanced, focused, and in control, no matter what challenges you face.

In small doses, stress can be a good thing. The stress response is the body's way of protecting you. When working properly, it helps you perform under pressure, rise to meet challenges, and stay focused, energetic, and alert. But beyond a certain point, stress stops being helpful and starts causing damage.

When stress is out-of-control, it can get in the way of your ability to:

- Think clearly and creatively
- Communicate clearly
- Accurately "read" other people
- Hear what someone is really saying
- Trust others
- Attend to your own needs

To assess your present ability to manage stress, ask yourself the following questions and answer 'yes', 'no', or ' rarely';

- When I feel agitated, do I know how to quickly calm myself?
- Can I easily let go of my anger?
- Can I turn to others at work to help me calm down and feel better?
- When I come home at night, do I walk in the door feeling alert and relaxed?
- Am I often distracted or moody?
- Am I able to recognize upsets that others seem to be experiencing?
- Do I easily turn to friends or family members for a calming influence?
- When my energy is low, do I know how to boost it?

If you answered 'yes' to most of these questions, you are probably in control of stress.

Signs that you may be stressed

- You feel drained and depleted
- You can't concentrate or think straight
- You feel nervous and keyed up
- Your stomach is upset
- You're having trouble sleeping
- Your muscles are tense
- You are continually irritable

If we don't know how to manage stressful situations in our lives, they can paralyse us emotionally and undermine even the strongest love or work relationships.

The first tip to managing stress is realizing when you're stressed and recognizing what stress feels like. Many of us spend so much time in a stressed state, we have forgotten what it feels like to be fully relaxed and alert. What does it feel like to be calm and stress-free? You can see that inner balance in the smile of a happy baby—a face so full of joy it reminds adults of the balanced emotional state that most of us have misplaced. In adulthood, being balanced means maintaining a calm state of energy, alertness, and focus. Calmness is more than just feeling relaxed; being alert is an equally important aspect of finding the balance needed to withstand stress.

The second tip to managing stress is to identify your stress response. Everyone reacts differently to stress. Some people get angry and do or say things they regret. Others shut down, withdraw, or freeze with anxiety. The best way to quickly relieve stress and calm yourself down depends on your specific stress response.

The most common ways people respond to stress are:

- An angry or agitated stress response. You're heated, keyed up, overly emotional, and unable to sit still.
- A withdrawn or depressed stress response. You shut down, space out, and show very little energy or emotion.
- A tense and frozen stress response. You freeze under pressure and can't do anything. You look paralysed, but under the surface you're extremely agitated.

When it comes to managing and reducing stress quickly in the middle of a heated situation, it's important to know whether you tend to become overexcited or under-excited when overwhelmed. If you tend to become angry, agitated, or keyed up under stress, you will respond best to stress-relief activities that are calming and soothing. If you tend to become frozen, depressed, withdrawn, or spaced-out under stress, you will respond best to stress relief activities that are stimulating and that energize your nervous system.

The third tip to managing and reducing stress is to discover what works for you. The best way to reduce stress quickly and reliably is through the senses: through sight, sound, smell, taste, and touch. Each person responds differently to these sensory inputs. You need to find things that are soothing to you. We all have different preferences and needs. What some people find soothing may be unpleasant or even stressful to others. For example, certain kinds of music may relax one person but irritate another. So you need to spend time figuring out what works for you. Then you can use what you've learned to create calming, sensory-rich environments at home, in your car, at the office, or wherever you spend time.

Knowing the right kind of sensory input is essential to:

- speed up, if you are a person who is spaced out or depressed when stressed.
- slow down, if you are a person who is angry or agitated when stressed
- to help get unstuck, if you are a person who is frozen with anxiety when stressed.

Understanding Stress
Modern life is full of hassles, deadlines, frustrations, and demands. For many people, stress is so commonplace that it has become a way of life. When you're constantly running in emergency mode, your mind and body pay the price. If you frequently find yourself feeling frazzled and overwhelmed, it's time to take action to bring your nervous system back into balance. You can protect yourself by learning how to recognize the signs and

symptoms of stress and taking steps to reduce its harmful effects.

When you perceive a threat, your nervous system responds by releasing a flood of stress hormones, including adrenaline and cortisol. These hormones rouse the body for emergency action. Your heart pounds faster, muscles tighten, blood pressure rises, breath quickens, and your senses become sharper. These physical changes increase your strength and stamina, speed your reaction time, and enhance your focus – preparing you to either fight or flee from the danger at hand. Stress is a normal physical response to events that make you feel threatened or that upset your balance in some way. When you sense danger – whether it's real or imagined – the body's defenses kick into high gear in a rapid, automatic process known as the "fight-or-flight" reaction, or the *stress response*. The stress response is the body's way of protecting you. When working properly, it helps you stay focused, energetic, and alert. In emergency situations, stress can save your life – giving you extra strength to defend yourself for example, or spurring you to slam on the brakes to avoid an accident.

The stress response also helps you rise to meet challenges. Stress is what keeps you on your toes during a presentation at work, sharpens your concentration when you're attempting the game-winning free throw, or drives you to study for an exam when you'd rather be socialising with your friends. But beyond a certain point, stress stops being helpful and starts causing major damage to your health, your mood, your productivity, your relationships, and your quality of life.

The body doesn't distinguish between physical and psychological threats. When you're stressed over a busy schedule, an argument with a friend, a traffic jam, or a mountain of bills, your body reacts just as strongly as if you were facing a life-or-death situation. If you have a lot of responsibilities and worries, your emergency stress response may be on most of the time. The more your body's stress system is activated the harder it is to shut off.

Long-term exposure to stress can lead to serious health problems. Chronic stress disrupts nearly every system in your body. It can raise blood pressure, suppress the immune system, increase the risk of heart attack and stroke. Long-term stress can even rewire the brain, leaving you more vulnerable to anxiety and depression. Many health problems are caused or exacerbated by stress, including:

- Pain of any kind
- High blood pressure
- Heart disease
- Digestive problems
- Sleep problems
- Depression
- Obesity
- Autoimmune diseases
- Skin conditions, such as eczema
- Back pain

Because of the widespread damage stress can cause, it's important to know your own limit. But just how much stress is too much, differs from person to person. Some people roll with the punches, while others crumble at the slightest obstacle or frustration. Some people even seem to thrive on the excitement and challenge of a high-stress lifestyle. Your ability to tolerate stress depends on many factors, including the quality of your relationships, your general outlook on life, your emotional intelligence, your life experience and genetics.

Your support network influences your stress tolerance. A strong network of supportive friends and family members is an enormous buffer against life's stressors. On the flip side, the more lonely and isolated you are, the greater your vulnerability to stress.

Your sense of control influences your stress tolerance. If you have confidence in yourself and your ability to influence events and persevere through challenges, it's easier to take stress in your stride. People who are vulnerable to stress tend to feel like things are out of their control.

Your attitude and outlook influences your stress tolerance. Stress-hardy people have an optimistic attitude. They tend to embrace challenges, have a strong sense of humour, accept that change is a part of life, and believe in a higher power or purpose.

Your ability to deal with your emotions influences your stress tolerance. You're extremely vulnerable to stress if you don't know how to calm and soothe yourself when you're feeling sad, angry, or afraid. The ability to bring your emotions into balance helps you bounce back from adversity.

Your knowledge and preparation influences your stress tolerance. The more you know about a stressful situation, including how long it will last and what to expect, the easier it is to cope. For example, if you go into surgery with a realistic picture of what to expect afterwards, a painful recovery will be less traumatic than if you were expecting to bounce back immediately.

Causes of stress
Stressful Life Events – not necessarily in any order. The level of stress in your life will depend on what the stress trigger means to you.

- Spouse's death
- Divorce
- Marriage separation
- Lack of Sleep
- Moving house
- Jail term
- Death of a close relative
- Injury or illness

- Relationship and Marriage difficulties
- Financial problems
- Redundancy, loss of a job
- Marriage reconciliation
- Retirement
- Work
- Too busy, lack of time
- Too many demands
- Time debting, giving all your time to others

The potential causes of stress are numerous and highly individual. What causes stress depends, at least in part, on your perception of it. Something that's stressful to you may not faze someone else; they may even enjoy it. For example, your morning commute may make you anxious and tense because you worry that traffic will make you late. Others, however, may find the trip relaxing because they allow more than enough time and enjoy listening to music while they drive.

The situations and pressures that cause stress are known as stressors. We usually think of stressors as being negative, such as an exhausting work schedule or a rocky relationship. However, anything that puts high demands on you or forces you to adjust can be stressful. This includes positive events such as getting married, buying a house, going to college, or receiving a promotion.

It's important to learn how to recognize when your stress levels are out of control. The most dangerous thing about stress is how easily it can creep up on you. You get used to it. It starts to feels familiar – even normal. You don't notice how much it's affecting you, even as it takes a heavy toll. The signs and symptoms of stress overload can be almost anything. Stress affects the mind, body, and behaviour in many ways, and everyone experiences stress differently.

Keep in mind that the signs and symptoms of stress can also be caused by other psychological and medical problems. If you're experiencing any of the warning signs of stress, it's important to see a doctor for a full evaluation. Your doctor can help you determine whether or not your symptoms are stress-related.

While unchecked stress is undeniably damaging, there are many things you can do to reduce its impact and cope with symptoms. You may feel like the stress in your life is out of your control, but you can always control the way you respond. Managing stress is all about taking charge: taking charge of your thoughts, your emotions, your schedule, your environment, and the way you deal with problems. Stress management involves changing the stressful situation when you can, changing your reaction when you can't, taking care of yourself, and making time for rest and relaxation.

A strong support network is your greatest protection against stress. When you have trusted friends and family members you know you can count on, life's pressures don't seem as overwhelming. So spend time with the people you love and don't let your responsibilities keep you from having a social life. If you don't have any close relationships, or your relationships *are* the source of your stress, make it a priority to build stronger and more satisfying connections.

Tips for reaching out and building relationships:

- Help someone else, become a volunteer
- Have lunch or coffee with a co-worker.
- Call or email an old friend.
- Go for a walk with a workout friend
- Schedule a weekly dinner date
- Take a class or join a club

Learning how to relax
You can't completely eliminate stress from your life, but you can control how much it affects you. Relaxation techniques such as yoga, meditation, and deep breathing activate the body's relaxation response, a state of restfulness that is the opposite of the stress response.

When practiced regularly, these activities lead to a reduction in your everyday stress levels and boost your feelings of joy and serenity. They also increase your ability to stay calm and collected under pressure.

Most people ignore their emotional health until there's a problem. But just as it requires time and energy to build or maintain your physical health, so it is with your emotional well-being. The more you put in to it, the stronger it will be. People with good emotional health have an ability to bounce back from stress and adversity. This ability is called resilience. They remain focused, flexible and positive in bad times as well as good. The good news is that there are many steps you can take to build your resilience and your overall emotional health.

Starting a relaxation practice
Learning the basics of a relaxation technique isn't difficult, however it takes daily practice to truly harness the stress-relieving power of these techniques. Most stress experts recommend setting aside at least ten to twenty minutes a day for your relaxation practice. If you'd like to get even more stress relief, aim for thirty minutes to an hour.

The best way to start and maintain a relaxation practice is by incorporating it into your daily routine. Schedule a set time either once or twice a day for your practice. You may find that it's easier to stick with your practice if you do it first thing in the morning, before other tasks and responsibilities get in the way. Don't practice when you're sleepy. These techniques can relax you so much that they can make you very sleepy, especially if it's close to bedtime. You will get the most out of these techniques if you practice when you're fully awake and alert. Choose a technique that appeals to you. There is no single relaxation technique that is best. When choosing a relaxation technique, consider your specific needs, preferences, and fitness level. The right relaxation technique is the one that resonates with you and fits your lifestyle. If you crave solitude, solo relaxation techniques such as meditation or progressive muscle relaxation will help you to quiet your mind and recharge your batteries. If you crave social interaction, a class setting will give you the stimulation and support you're looking for. Practicing with others may also help you stay motivated.

Using the five senses to quickly relieve and manage stress
Learning the sensory stress-busting techniques that work for you gives you a powerful tool for staying clear-headed and in control. You'll have the confidence to face challenges, knowing that you have the ability to rapidly bring yourself back into a state of equilibrium.

It's important to identify stress relief techniques that:

- Both relax and energize you
- Have an immediate impact on your stress
- Are enjoyable and make you feel good
- Consistently work for you
- Are always available or easily accessible

You can rapidly reverse the effects of stress by exposing yourself to sensory input that brings you back into balance. Sensory input encompasses what we hear, feel, touch, taste, and see. You can use the five senses to soothe, comfort, and invigorate yourself almost immediately.

Try out these six stress-busting techniques and see what works best for you:

1.   Movement for quick stress relief
If you tend to shut down when you're under stress, stress-relieving activities that get you moving may be particularly helpful. Anything that engages the muscles or gets you up and active can work. Here are a few suggestions:

- Run in place
- Jump up and down
- Dance around

- Roll your head in circles
- Do a few quick yoga stretches
- Stomp your feet
- Go for a short walk
- Squeeze a rubbery stress ball
- Do some shadow boxing

2.   Sight for quick stress relief

If you're a visual person, try to manage and relieve stress by surrounding yourself with soothing and uplifting images. You can also try closing your eyes and visualising soothing images. Here are a few visually-based activities that may work as quick stress relievers:

- Decorate your home or office with cherished photos and favourite mementos.
- Bring the outside indoors; buy a plant or some flowers to enliven your space.
- Enjoy the beauty of nature—a garden, the beach, a park, or your own backyard.
- Surround yourself with colours that lift your spirits (paint your walls with your favourite colour, for example)
- Close your eyes and picture a situation or place that feels peaceful and rejuvenating (e.g. playing with a beloved pet or baby; enjoying a game of tennis or basketball; a day at the seashore swimming in clear blue water). The more sensory-rich the image, the better.

3.   Touch for quick stress relief

Experiment with your sense of touch, playing with different tactile sensations. Focus on things you can feel that are relaxing and renewing. Use the following suggestions as a starting point:

- Wrap yourself in a warm blanket.
- Pet a dog or cat.
- Hold a comforting object or a favourite memento.
- Soak in a hot bath.
- Give yourself a hand or neck massage.

- Wear clothing that feels soft against your skin.

4. Sound for quick stress relief

Are you sensitive to sounds and noises? Are you a music lover? If so, stress-relieving exercises that focus on your auditory sense may work particularly well. Experiment with the following sounds, noting how quickly your stress levels drop as you listen:

- Sing or a hum a favourite tune.
- Listen to uplifting music.
- Tune in to the soundtrack of nature–crashing waves, the wind rustling the trees, birds singing.
- Play an instrumental or classical CD.
- Hang wind chimes near an open window.
- Buy a small fountain, so you can enjoy the soothing sound of running water in your home or office.

5. Smell for quick stress relief

If you tend to zone out or freeze when stressed, surround yourself with smells that are energizing and invigorating. If you tend to become overly agitated under stress, look for scents that are comforting and calming.

- Spray on your favourite perfume or cologne.
- Light a scented candle or burn some incense.
- Lie down in sheets scented with lavender.
- Breathe in the smell of freshly brewed coffee or tea.
- Smell some roses or another type of scented flower.
- Enjoy the clean, fresh air in the great outdoors.

6. Taste for quick stress relief

Slowly savouring a favourite treat can be very relaxing, but mindless stress eating will only add to your stress and your waistline. The key is to indulge your sense of taste mindfully and in moderation.

- Eat slowly, focusing on the feel of the food in your mouth and the taste on your tongue:
- Drink a refreshing cold beverage.
- Chew a piece of sugarless gum.

- Indulge in a small piece of dark chocolate.
- Sip a steaming cup of tea.
- Enjoy a perfectly ripe piece of fruit.
- Savour a healthy, crunchy snack. Try celery, carrots, or fruit mix.

Learning to use your senses to quickly manage stress is a little like learning to drive or to play golf. You don't master the skill in one lesson–you have to practice until it becomes second nature. Once you have a variety of sensory tools which you can depend on and use, you will be able to handle even the toughest of situations.

Relaxation techniques for stress-relief

The following are some relaxation techniques that you can call upon:

1. Deep breathing for stress relief
2. Progressive muscle relaxation for stress relief
3. Mindfulness meditation for stress relief
4. Guided imagery for stress relief
5. Yoga for stress relief
6. Tai chi for stress relief
7. Massage therapy for stress relief

1.Deep breathing for stress relief
With its focus on full, cleansing breaths, deep breathing is a simple, yet powerful, relaxation technique. It's easy to learn, can be practiced almost anywhere, and provides a quick way to get your stress levels in check. Deep breathing is the cornerstone of many other relaxation practices and can be combined with other relaxing elements such as aromatherapy and music.

The key to deep breathing is to breathe deeply from the abdomen, getting as much fresh air as possible in your lungs. When you take deep breaths from the abdomen, rather than shallow breaths from your upper chest, you inhale more oxygen. The more oxygen you get, the less tense, short of breath, and anxious you feel. So the next time you feel stressed, take a minute to slow down and breathe deeply:

- Sit comfortably with your back straight. Put one hand on your chest and the other on your stomach.
- Breathe in through your nose. The hand on your stomach should rise. The hand on your chest should move very little.
- Exhale through your mouth, pushing out as much air as you can while contracting your abdominal muscles. The hand on your stomach should move in

as you exhale, but your other hand should move very little.
- Continue to breathe in through your nose and out through your mouth. Try to inhale enough so that your lower abdomen rises and falls. Count slowly as you exhale.
- If you have a hard time breathing from your abdomen while sitting up, try lying on the floor. Put a small book on your stomach, and try to breathe so that the book rises as you inhale and falls as you exhale.

2.   Progressive muscle relaxation for stress relief
Progressive muscle relaxation is another effective and widely used technique for stress relief. It involves a two-step process in which you systematically tense and relax different muscle groups in the body. With regular practice, progressive muscle relaxation gives you an intimate familiarity with how tension, as well as complete relaxation, feels in different parts of the body. This awareness helps you spot and counteract the first signs of the muscular tension that accompanies stress. And as your body relaxes, so will your mind. You can combine deep breathing with progressive muscle relaxation for an additional level of relief from stress.

Progressive Muscle Relaxation Sequence:
- Right foot
- Left foot
- Right calf
- Left calf
- Right thigh
- Left thigh
- Hips and buttocks
- Stomach
- Chest
- Back
- Right arm and hand
- Left arm and hand
- Neck and shoulders
- Face

Most progressive muscle relaxation practitioners start at the feet and work their way up to the face.

Loosen your clothing, take off your shoes, and get comfortable. Take a few minutes to relax, breathing in and out in slow, deep breaths. When you're relaxed and ready to start, shift your attention to your right foot. Take a moment to focus on the way it feels. Slowly tense the muscles in your right foot, squeezing as tightly as you can. Hold for a count of ten. Relax your right foot. Focus on the tension flowing away and the way your foot feels as it becomes limp and loose. Stay in this relaxed state for a moment, breathing deeply and slowly. When you're ready, shift your attention to your left foot. Follow the same sequence of muscle tension and release. Move slowly up through your body — legs, abdomen, back, neck, face — contracting and relaxing the muscle groups as you go. When you have tensed and relaxed all the muscle groups, take a few moments to enjoy the feeling of total body relaxation.

3.   Mindfulness meditation for stress relief
Meditation that cultivates mindfulness is particularly effective at reducing stress, anxiety, depression, and other negative emotions. Mindfulness is the quality of being fully engaged in the present moment, in the now, without analysing or otherwise over-thinking the experience. Rather than worrying about the future or dwelling on the past, mindfulness meditation switches the focus to what's happening right now.

For stress relief, try the following mindfulness meditation techniques:

Body scan – Body scanning cultivates mindfulness by focusing your attention on various parts of your body. Like progressive muscle relaxation, you start with your feet and work your way up. However, instead of tensing and relaxing your muscles, you simply focus on the way each part of your body feels without labelling the sensations as either "good" or "bad".

Walking meditation - You don't have to be seated or still to meditate. In walking meditation, mindfulness involves being focused on the physicality of each step — the sensation of your feet touching the ground, the rhythm of your breath while moving, and feeling the wind against your face.

Mindful eating – If you reach for food when you're under stress or gulp your meals down in a rush, try eating mindfully. Sit down at the table and focus your full attention on the meal (no TV, newspapers, or eating on the run). Eat slowly, taking the time to fully enjoy and savour each bite.

Mindfulness meditation is not equal to zoning out. It takes effort to maintain your concentration and to bring it back to the present moment when your mind wanders or you start to drift off. But with regular practice, mindfulness meditation strengthens the areas of the brain associated with joy and relaxation, and weakens those involved in negativity and stress.

4.   Guided imagery for stress relief
Visualization, or guided imagery, is a variation on traditional meditation that can help relieve stress. When used as a relaxation technique, guided imagery involves imagining a scene in which you feel at peace, free to let go of all tension and anxiety. Choose whatever setting is most calming to you, whether a tropical beach, a favourite childhood spot, or a quiet wooded glen. You can do this visualization exercise on your own, with a therapist's help, or using an audio recording.   Close your eyes and let your worries drift away. Imagine your restful place. Picture it as vividly as you can—everything you can see, hear, smell, and feel. Guided imagery works best if you incorporate as many sensory details as possible. For example, if you are thinking about a place beside a quiet lake:

- **See** the sun setting over the water
- **Hear** the birds singing
- **Smell** the pine trees
- **Feel** the cool water on your bare feet
- **Taste** the fresh, clean air

5.   Yoga for stress relief

Yoga is an excellent stress relief technique. It involves a series of both moving and stationary poses, combined with deep breathing. The physical and mental benefits of yoga provide a natural counterbalance to stress, and strengthen the relaxation response in your daily life.

Although almost all yoga classes end in a relaxation pose, classes that emphasize slow, steady movement and gentle stretching are best for stress relief. Look for labels like *gentle,* for *stress relief,* or for *beginners.* Power yoga, with its intense poses and focus on fitness, is not the best choice. If you're unsure whether a specific yoga class is appropriate for stress relief, call the studio or ask the teacher. Since injuries can happen when yoga is practiced incorrectly, it's best to learn by attending group classes or hiring a private teacher. Once you've learned the basics, you can practice alone or with others, tailoring your practice as you see fit.

Consider your fitness level and any medical issues before joining a yoga class. There are many yoga classes for different needs, such as prenatal yoga, yoga for seniors, and adaptive yoga (modified yoga for disabilities). Look for a low-pressure environment where you can learn at your own pace. Don't extend yourself beyond what feels comfortable, and always stop at the first sign of pain. A good teacher can show you alternative poses for ones that are too challenging for your health or fitness level.

6.   Tai chi for stress relief

If you've ever seen a group of people in the park slowly moving in synch, you've probably witnessed Tai Chi. Tai Chi is a self-paced, non-competitive series of slow, flowing body movements. These movements emphasize concentration, relaxation, and the conscious circulation of vital energy throughout the body. Though Tai Chi has its roots in martial arts, today it is primarily practiced as a way of calming the mind, conditioning the body, and reducing stress. As in meditation, Tai Chi practitioners focus on their breathing and keeping their attention in the present moment. Tai Chi is a safe, low-impact option for people of all ages and levels of fitness, including older adults and those recovering from injuries. Once you've learned the moves, you can practice it anywhere, at any time, by yourself, or with others.

As with yoga, Tai Chi is best learned in a class or from a private instructor. Although Tai Chi is normally very safe and gentle, be sure to discuss any health or mobility concerns with your instructor.

7.   Massage therapy for stress relief
Getting a massage provides deep relaxation, and as the muscles in your body relax, so does your overstressed mind. You don't have to visit the spa to enjoy the benefits of massage. There are many simple self-massage techniques you can use to relax and release stress.

Self Massage Techniques:

Scalp Soother
Place your thumbs behind your ears while spreading your fingers on top of your head. Move your scalp back and forth slightly by making circles with your fingertips for 15-20 seconds.

Easy on the Eyes
Close your eyes and place your ring fingers directly under your eyebrows, near the bridge of your nose. Slowly and gently increase the pressure on this area for 5-10 seconds, then gently release. Repeat 2-3 times

Shoulder Tension Relief

Reach one arm across the front of your body to your opposite shoulder. Using a circular motion, press firmly on the muscle above your shoulder blade. Repeat on the other side

The most common type of massage is Swedish massage, a soothing technique specifically designed to relax and energize. Another common type of massage is Shiatsu, also known as acupressure. In Shiatsu massage, therapists use their fingers to manipulate the body's pressure points. Although self-massage is good for stress relief, getting a massage from a professional massage therapist can be tremendously relaxing and more beneficial than what you can do yourself. When booking a massage, try types like Swedish or Shiatsu, which promote overall relaxation. Deep tissue and sports massages are more aggressive. They often target specific areas and may leave you sore for a couple of days, making them less effective for relaxation and stress relief.

*

Remember, your ability to manage stress allows you to remain emotionally available to others, to communicate clearly and stay balanced no matter what challenges you face.

Skill Two - The ability to manage your emotions

The second skill for building rewarding and lasting relationships is the ability to recognize and manage your emotions. Emotional exchanges hold the communication process together. To communicate in a way that grabs or engages others, you have to be able to access your emotions and recognize how they influence your actions and relationships. However, your emotions may be distorted, numbed, or buried – especially if you've experienced early-life traumas such as loss, isolation, or abuse. Unfortunately, without emotional awareness, we are unable to fully understand our own motivations and needs, or to communicate effectively with others. In order to be emotionally healthy and emotionally intelligent, you must reconnect to your core emotions.

Managing and Dealing with Your Emotions and Feelings

Emotions connect people to one another. They are the foundation of your ability to understand yourself and relate to others. When you are aware and in control of your emotions, you can think clearly and creatively; manage stress and challenges; communicate well with others; and display trust, empathy, and confidence. But lose control of your emotions, and you'll spin into confusion, isolation, and doubt. By learning to recognize, manage, and deal with your emotions, you'll enjoy greater happiness and health and better relationships.

As an infant, your emotions connected you to your primary caregiver in what was the first relationship of your life. Throughout life, emotions continue to serve this same purpose: connecting you to others.

Your emotions help you to:

- understand yourself, including your deeply-felt needs
- understand and empathize with others
- communicate clearly and effectively

- make decisions based on the things that are most important to you
- get motivated and take action to meet goals
- build strong, healthy relationships

Whether you're having an argument with your spouse or dealing with colleagues at work, your emotions influence the communication process. Over ninety five percent of communication is nonverbal and emotionally driven, so the stakes in learning to harness your emotions are high. Say the wrong thing, or miss an emotional cue, and it can cause a lot of damage.

Evaluating your emotional awareness
Although emotional awareness is the basis of emotional health, good communication, and solid relationships, many people remain relatively unacquainted with their core emotional experience. It is surprising how few people can easily answer the question: "What are you experiencing emotionally?"

Emotional awareness involves two basic abilities:

- The ability to recognize your moment-to-moment emotional experience
- The ability to manage all of your feelings appropriately

What is your level of emotional awareness?
Ask yourself the following questions. If you can answer "yes" to most of the questions, congratulations! If not, you may want to work on raising your emotional awareness:

- Can you tolerate strong feelings, including anger, sadness, fear, disgust, and joy?
- Do you feel your emotions in your body? If you are sad or mad, do you experience physical sensations in places like your stomach, chest or shoulders?

- Are you comfortable with all of your emotions? No one chooses to be angry, sad or frightened but if you are, is it OK?
- Do you pay attention to your emotions and use them to guide your decisions?
- Are you comfortable talking about your emotions? Do you communicate your feelings honestly?
- Do your emotions capture the attention of others?
- Do others know what you feel? Are you comfortable with their knowing?
- Are you sensitive to the emotions of others?

We are all born with a capacity to freely experience the full range of human emotions, including joy, anger, sadness, and fear. Yet many people are disconnected from some or all of their feelings. By trying to avoid pain and discomfort, their emotions have become distorted, displaced, and stifled.

You may avoid strong emotions you fear or dislike by distracting yourself with obsessive thoughts, escapist fantasies, mindless entertainment, and addictive behaviours. Watching television for hours, playing computer games, and surfing the Internet are common ways of avoiding dealing with feelings. Another avoidance method is sticking with one emotional response that you feel comfortable with, no matter what the situation calls for. For example: constantly joking around to cover up insecurities or getting angry all the time to avoid feeling frightened and sad. If you feel overwhelmed by your emotions, you may cope by numbing yourself and shutting down or shutting out intense emotions. You may feel completely disconnected from your emotions, as if you no longer have feelings at all.

The consequences of avoiding emotions and feelings

You lose the good, along with the bad. You either feel your emotions or you don't. When you shut down negative feelings like anger, fear, or sadness, you also shut down your ability to experience positive feelings such as joy, love, and happiness. It's exhausting. You can distort and numb emotions, but you can't eliminate them entirely. It takes a lot of energy to avoid having an authentic emotional experience and keep your feelings suppressed. The effort leaves you stressed and drained. It damages your relationships. The more you distance yourself from your feelings, the more distant you become from others, as well as yourself. You lose the ability to build strong relationships and communicate effectively, both of which depend on being in touch with your own emotions.

Remember you can't manage emotions until you know how to manage stress. The ability to manage stress is a prerequisite for emotional awareness. Raising your emotional awareness and emotional intelligence begins with the question: "What kinds of sensory input instantly makes me feel relaxed, safe, calm, and focused?" Knowing the answer is especially important for people who have had overwhelming emotional experiences as a child. Once you have a safety net in place and know how to make yourself feel good quickly and dependably, you can begin to explore the emotions that seem disagreeable or frightening. The key to coping with strong emotions is knowing that you control them, not the other way around.

The ability to quickly reduce stress allows you to safely face strong emotions, secure in your ability to regulate your feelings and behave appropriately. When you know how to maintain a relaxed, energized state of awareness— even when something upsetting happens, you can remain emotionally available and engaged.

Getting back in touch with your emotions and feelings

The process of raising emotional awareness involves reconnecting with all of the core emotions, including anger, sadness, fear, disgust, surprise, and joy.

As you start this process, keep the following facts about emotions and emotional awareness in mind; emotions quickly come and go, if we let them. You may be worried that once you reconnect to the emotions you've been avoiding, you'll be stuck with them forever, but that's not so. When we don't stoke our emotions with thoughts about them, even the most painful and difficult feelings subside and lose their power to control our attention.

Unrestricted, the core emotions of anger, sadness, fear, and joy quickly come and go. Throughout the day, you'll see, read, or hear something that momentarily triggers a strong feeling of some sort. If you don't focus on the feeling, it won't last, and a different emotion will soon take its place.

Our bodies can clue us in to our emotions. Our emotions are closely aligned to physical sensations in our bodies. When you experience a strong emotion, you should also feel it somewhere in your body. By paying attention to these physical sensations, you can understand your emotions better

You don't have to choose between thinking and feeling. Once you have confidence in your ability to safely experience any of your emotions, you can think, plan, and engage in a wide range of intellectual activities without completely losing touch with the physical sensations in your body that signal your emotional state.

Emotional awareness can be a background condition that functions like instinct. When it's strongly developed, you'll know what you are feeling without having to think about it. When your emotional signals become strong enough, you realize that something important is going on and you can shift your focus accordingly.

How to raise your emotional awareness

The key to raising emotional awareness is practice. Like building muscles in a gym, the more you flex your emotions, the more emotional muscle you'll build. You wouldn't expect to be a bodybuilder after just five minutes. The more consistently you practice, the greater the change you'll experience in what you feel, think, and do. To develop your self-awareness and your connection to others and incorporate it into your life, you need to retrain yourself through hands-on exercises and real-world practice.

How will you know when you have practiced enough? In general you should feel more energy, experience more positive feelings and have a greater ability to concentrate your attention. You should feel more alive!

Developing emotional awareness skills

When you started to ride a bike you probably used stabilizers or an older sibling to hold on to you. This helped you overcome your fear of falling until you gradually developed trust in your natural sense of balance, and experienced the joy of a new way of moving in the world. The process of learning to ride the waves of your emotions can touch on some feelings that may be painful and fearful. It's recommended that you have first practiced and learned some of the earlier stress relief techniques. These are the stabilizers that make riding the emotional waves feel comfortable and less fearful. Have these tools available at all times. Be very familiar with your typical response to stress and the sensory means that you find both calming and balancing.

To start developing emotional awareness skills, pick a time well before bedtime, so you won't fall asleep. Establish an environment of sensory support. Find a private spot that meets your sensory needs, one where your surroundings feel completely safe and comfortable. Take off your shoes and loosen your belt or any tight clothing. Take the phone off the hook, and close the door.

Find a comfortable chair that supports your back, or lie down (but only if you're sure you won't drift off to sleep). Don't smoke, drink alcohol, or eat during this process.

If this is your first time, try allocating fifteen minutes to this part of the process. Tense, tighten, and then release each part of your body. You can work from your feet up to the top of your head, or you can do it in whatever order feels right for you. Squeeze each body part for a count of five seconds before releasing, and then allow each part to feel completely limp and relaxed. Clear your mind of extraneous thoughts. Close your eyes and take several slow, deep breaths, releasing your thoughts each time you exhale.

Make sure to exhale as much air as you inhaled. Put one hand on your chest and the other on your belly. Are both of your hands moving? If not, breathe in a little more fully and exhale a little more completely. As you continue, allow your body to sink comfortably into the chair or floor. It's not easy to clear your mind of thoughts, but when unwanted thoughts intermittently pop back into your consciousness, focus on your breathing. Try to let go of those thoughts while exhaling.

For the first session, choose an emotional trigger (anger, sadness or fear) that had a moderate emotional effect on you (e.g., maybe someone was rude or cut in front of you). What you choose can be either an emotional memory or a feeling you are still experiencing. Slowly scan your entire body to find the spot where a feeling is most intense. Is it in your stomach, chest, shoulders, or somewhere else? Focus all of your attention on this one area and direct your breath to its core. Experience the physical sensations that occur while you continue to breathe deeply.

Again, allow the feelings to take root by continuing to breathe deeply into the area where you experience the greatest intensity. You are trying to bring a fuzzy feeling into focus. At other times, these sensations are accompanied by visual memories. Everyone's experience is unique. If you become too uncomfortable, redirect your focus to a sensory input that is calming and balancing – your stress-control tool kit. Indulge these pleasant feelings until you feel safe and comfortable. When you're ready, go back into the uncomfortable feelings you were exploring. Pivot back and forth as often as necessary until your allotted time is up, then seamlessly switch back to the world around you.

Every time you correctly practice the exercise, you should feel a little more in control of your feelings.

To connect with more intense emotions, wait until you are familiar and comfortable with the earlier exercise before doing this. As you become comfortable experiencing moderately intense emotions, you can move in to focus on increasingly intense feelings. Remember, if you become sufficiently uncomfortable, toggle back and forth between the feelings and the sensory input. You may begin with one feeling, but find that soon it shifts into another feeling or that the source of the feeling moves from one location in your body to a different place. Follow the new feeling as long as it proves to be more intense than the last. If you're not experiencing much feeling of any sort, focus on just that – what it feels like to feel nothing. Hang in there. Try to stay with the most intense feeling for as long as you can. Remember the goal is not emotional release; it's emotional integration. Don't force the issue and push for a release; a bit at a time is just as effective and less taxing. The point here is to allow rather than force the feelings to emerge. This process is about trusting your body to indicate how much it wants you to feel in this moment. You'll get better at it over time. Some people cry during this part of the process, but not necessarily due to sadness. If they've been repressing feelings for a long time, the release can be intense. But tears are not necessary for a release. Some people moan or make other sounds, sometimes stretching or spontaneously moving their bodies during the process.

Trembling is common and a natural part of releasing and rebalancing after a traumatic experience – your mind may be saying an intense feeling is not okay. Just remind yourself that it is okay. So if you begin to tremble, continue to breathe deeply and hold your focus. You can always switch to one of the relaxation techniques from your stress-relieving tool kit.

When your allotted time is finished, seamlessly switch back to the world around you. The purpose of this part is to integrate the process and empower you with a greater sense of mastery and control of your emotions. Get up, open your eyes wide and stretch. Stamp your feet, move your body, and walk around. Congratulate yourself for completing such an intense exercise. Stop focusing exclusively on your feelings, and redirect your thoughts toward your normal daily activities. Although your focus has now shifted from your inner world back to your outer life, you will retain some of the emotional awareness you just experienced. Take stock of your energy and focus. Notice whether colours seem brighter and sounds seem clearer.

To deepen the learning process and to integrate this skill into your life, find someone to share your experience. Within thirty six hours of performing this exercise, find someone who is a good listener and share your experience of this process with him or her. Talking about your emotional experience helps reinforce and integrate the new learning.

Practice the exercise often. Practice until you feel comfortably in control of your emotional experiences. Remember, like building muscles in a gym, the more you flex emotions, the more "emotional muscle" you build.

Skill Three - The ability to communicate nonverbally

The third skill for building rewarding and lasting relationships is the ability to communicate nonverbally. The most powerful forms of communication contain no words, and take place at a much faster rate than speech. Using nonverbal communication is the way to attract other's attention and keep relationships on track. Eye contact, facial expression, tone of voice, posture, gesture, touch, intensity, timing, pace, and sounds that convey understanding engage the brain and influence others much more than your words alone. The way we talk, listen, look, and move will produce a sense of interest, trust, excitement and desire for connection – or they will generate fear, confusion, distrust and disinterest.

Nonverbal communication isn't about words, but it's not necessarily silent; tone of voice or a well-placed sigh can say a great deal. And, it is a visual language. If a conversationalist is standing stiffly, the message he sends may be quite different than if he is visibly relaxed. An obvious eye-roll or a subtle shrug can speak volumes— even without the person's conscious intention. So, nonverbal communication is vital to keeping our relationships strong and healthy.

Part of improving our non-verbal communication involves paying attention to: eye contact, facial expression, tone of voice, posture, gestures and touch. Nonverbal communication consciously or unconsciously sends either positive or negative signals to others. Nothing reveals more to others about us, or attracts others to us, than wordless communication.

Nonverbal communication cues can play five roles:

- Repetition: they can repeat the message the person is making verbally
- Contradiction: they can contradict a message the individual is trying to convey

- Substitution: they can substitute for a verbal message. For example, a person's eyes can often convey a far more vivid message than words and often do
- Complementing: they may add to or complement a verbal message.
- Accenting: they may accent or underline a verbal message. Pounding the table, for example, would certainly underline a message.

Nonverbal communication and body language in relationships

It takes more than words to create fulfilling, strong relationships. Nonverbal communication has a huge impact on the quality of our relationships. Nonverbal communication skills improve relationships by helping you to:

- Accurately read other people, including the emotions they're feeling and the unspoken messages they're sending.
- Create trust and transparency in relationships by sending nonverbal signals that match up with your words.
- Respond with nonverbal cues that show others that you understand, notice, and care.

Unfortunately, many people send confusing or negative nonverbal signals without even knowing it. When this happens, both connection and trust are lost in our relationships.

Types of non-verbal communication

There are many different types of nonverbal communication. Together, the following nonverbal signals and cues communicate your interest and investment in others.

Facial expressions
The human face is extremely expressive, able to express countless emotions without saying a word. And unlike some forms of nonverbal communication, facial

expressions are universal. The facial expressions for happiness, sadness, anger, surprise, fear, and disgust are the same across cultures.

Body movements and posture
Consider how your perceptions of people are affected by the way they sit, walk, slouch, stand up straight, or hold their head. Likewise, the way you move and carry yourself communicates a wealth of information to the world.

Gestures
Gestures are woven into the fabric of our daily lives. We wave, point, beckon, and use our hands when we're arguing or speaking animatedly–expressing ourselves with gestures often without thinking. However, the meaning of gestures can be very different across cultures and regions, so it's important to be careful to avoid misinterpretation.

Eye contact
Since the visual sense is dominant for most people, eye contact is an especially important type of nonverbal communication. The way you look at someone can communicate many things, including interest, affection, hostility, or attraction. Eye contact is also important in maintaining the flow of conversation and for gauging the other person's response. However staring can be threatening and makes people feel uncomfortable.

Touch
We communicate a great deal through touch. Think about the messages given by the following: a firm handshake, a timid tap on the shoulder, a warm bear hug, a reassuring pat on the back, a patronizing pat on the head, or a controlling grip on the arm.

Space
Have you ever felt uncomfortable during a conversation because the other person was standing too close and invading your space? We all have a need for physical space, although that need differs depending on the culture, the situation, and the closeness of the

relationship. You can use physical space to communicate many different nonverbal messages, including signals of intimacy, aggression, dominance, or affection.

Voice
We communicate with our voices, even when we are not using words. Nonverbal speech sounds such as tone, pitch, volume, inflection, rhythm, and rate are important communication elements. When we speak, other people read our voices in addition to listening to our words. These nonverbal speech sounds provide subtle but powerful clues into our true feelings and what we really mean. Think about how the tone of your voice, for example, can indicate sarcasm, anger, affection, or confidence. It's not only what you say, it's how you say it!

Nonverbal communication is a rapidly flowing back-and-forth process. Successful nonverbal communication depends on emotional self-awareness and an understanding of the cues you're sending, along with the ability to accurately pick up on the cues others are sending you. This requires your full concentration and attention. If you are planning what you're going to say next, daydreaming, or thinking about something else, you are almost certain to miss nonverbal cues and other subtleties in the conversation. You need to stay focused on the moment-to-moment experience in order to fully understand what's going on.

Tips for successful nonverbal communication:

Take a time out if you're feeling overwhelmed by stress. Stress compromises your ability to communicate. When you're stressed out, you're more likely to misread other people, send off confusing or off-putting nonverbal signals, and lapse into unhealthy knee-jerk patterns of behaviour. Take a moment to calm down before you jump back into the conversation. Once you've regained your emotional equilibrium, you'll be better equipped to deal with the situation in a positive way.

Pay attention to inconsistencies. Nonverbal communication should reinforce what is being said. If you get the feeling that someone isn't being honest or that something is "off," you may be picking up on a mismatch between verbal and nonverbal cues. Is the person saying one thing, and their body language saying something else?

Look at nonverbal communication signals as a group. Don't read too much into a single gesture or nonverbal cue. Consider all of the nonverbal signals you are sending and receiving, from eye contact to tone of voice and body language. Do they all seem to be saying the same thing or hitting the same emotional mark?

Remember, most people instinctively send and interpret nonverbal signals all the time, so don't assume you're the only one who's aware of nonverbal undercurrents. Finally, stay true to yourself. Be aware of your own natural style, and don't adopt behaviour that is incompatible with it. Thinking you can bluff by deliberately altering your body language can do more harm than good. Unless you're a proficient actor, it will be hard to overcome your body's inability to lie. There will always be mixed messages, signs that your channels of communication are not congruent. It's something others will detect, one way or another.

Incorrect accusations based on erroneous observations can be embarrassing and damaging and take a long time to overcome. Always verify your interpretation with another communications channel before rushing in. You could say something like, "I get the feeling you're uncomfortable with this course of action. Would you like to add something to the discussion?" This should draw out the real message and force the individual to come clean or to adjust his or her body language.

Improving your nonverbal communication skills

Before you can improve your nonverbal communication skills, you need to figure out what you're doing right and where there is room for improvement.

These are some methods to observe yourself in action:

Video camera – Videotape a conversation between you and a partner. Set the camera to record both of you at the same time, so you can observe the nonverbal back-and-forth. When you watch the recording, focus on any discrepancies between your verbal and nonverbal communication.

Digital camera – Ask someone to take a series of photos of you while you're talking to someone else. As you look through the photos, focus on you and the other person's body language, facial expressions, and gestures.

Audio recorder – Record a conversation between you and a friend or family member. As you listen to the recording afterwards, concentrate on the way things are said, rather than the words. Pay attention to tone, timing, pace, and other sounds.

As you watch or listen to the recordings, ask yourself the following questions:

Eye contact
Is this source of connection missing, too intense, or just right in yourself or the person you are looking at?

Facial expression
What is your face showing? Is it mask-like and inexpressive, or emotionally present and filled with interest? What do you see as you look into the faces of others?

Tone of voice
Does your voice project warmth, confidence, and delight, or is it strained and blocked? What do you hear as you listen to other people?

Posture and gesture
Does your body feel still and immobile, or relaxed?
Sensing the degree of tension in your shoulders and jaw
answers this question. What do you observe about the
degree of tension or relaxation in the body of the person
you are speaking to?

Touch
Remember, what feels good is relative. How do you like to
be touched? Who do you like to have touching you? Is the
difference between what you like and what the other
person likes obvious to you?

Intensity
Do you or the person you are communicating with seem
flat, cool, and disinterested, or over-the-top and
melodramatic? Again, this has as much to do with what
feels good to the other person as it does with what you
personally prefer.

Timing and pace
What happens when you or someone you care about
makes an important statement? Does a response–not
necessarily verbal–come too quickly or too slowly? Is
there an easy flow of information back and forth?

Sounds
Do you use sounds to indicate that you are attending to
the other person? Do you pick up on sounds from others
that indicate their caring or concern for you?

The point of this exercise is to develop your nonverbal
awareness. As you continue to pay attention to the
nonverbal cues and signals you send and receive, your
ability to communicate will improve.

Skill Four - The ability to use humour and play

The fourth skill for building lasting and rewarding relationships is the ability to use humour and play in your relationships. Playfulness and humour help you navigate and rise above difficult and embarrassing issues. Mutually shared positive experiences also uplift you. They help you find inner resources needed to cope with disappointment and heartbreak, and give you the will to maintain a positive connection to your work and your loved ones.

Using playful communication in your relationships helps you to take hardships in your stride. By allowing you to view your frustrations and disappointments from new perspectives, laughter and play enable you to survive annoyances, hard times, and setbacks. Using gentle humour often helps you to say things that might be difficult without creating a bigger issue. Play relaxes your body and recharges your emotional batteries.

The Power of Laughter, Humour, and Play
Laughter has a powerful effect on your health and well-being. A good laugh relieves tension and stress, elevates mood, enhances creativity and problem-solving ability, and provides a quick energy boost. But even more importantly, laughter brings people together. Mutual laughter and play are an essential component of strong, healthy relationships. By making a conscious effort to incorporate more humour and play into your daily interactions, you can improve the quality of your loving relationships— as well as your connections with co-workers, family members, and friends.

Shared laughter is one of the most effective tools for keeping relationships exciting, fresh, and vital. Humour and playful communication strengthens our relationships by making us feel good and fostering emotional connection. People are attracted to happy, funny individuals. Laughter draws others to you and keeps them by your side.

When we laugh with one another, a positive bond is created. This bond acts as a strong buffer against stress, disagreements, and disappointment. And laughter really is contagious—just hearing laughter primes our brain and readies us to smile and join in on the fun. Humour, laughter, and play enrich our interactions and give our relationships that extra zing that keeps them exciting, light, and joyful. This shared pleasure creates a sense of intimacy and connection— qualities that define solid, lasting relationships.

Playful communication helps you:

- Smooth over differences. Using gentle humour often helps you broach sensitive subjects, resolve disagreements, and reframe problems.
- Feel relaxed and energized at the same time. Laughter relieves fatigue and relaxes your body, while also recharging your batteries and enabling you to accomplish more.
- Overcome problems and setbacks. A sense of humour is the key to resilience. It helps you take hardships in stride, weather disappointment, and bounce back from adversity and loss.

The health benefits of laughter
Laughter is a powerful tool when it comes to strengthening and maintaining both your physical and mental health.

Laughter bolsters your physical health by:

- Decreasing stress hormones
- Improving the flow of oxygen to the brain
- Reducing physical pain
- Lowering blood pressure
- Strengthening the immune system

The mental health benefits of laughter are tied to the physical benefits. When your body is relaxed and energized, you are better able to think and communicate clearly. This helps you keep your own emotions in check, relate in a positive way to others, and resolve conflict. Laughter is a particularly powerful antidote to depression and anxiety.

Having a sense of humour offsets depression and anxiety by:

- Releasing endorphins. When you laugh, your brain releases endorphins, powerful chemicals that boost mood and override sadness and negative thoughts.
- Putting things into perspective. Most situations are not as bleak as they appear to be when looked at from a playful and humorous point of view.
- Connecting us to others. Our mental health depends, to a large degree, on the quality of our relationships—and laughter binds people together.

Humour and playfulness strengthens relationships—but only when both people are in on the joke. It's important to be sensitive to the other person. If your partner, friend, or colleague isn't likely to appreciate the joke, don't say or do it, even if it's "all in good fun." When playfulness is one-sided rather than mutual, it undermines trust and goodwill and damages the relationship.

Playful communication in relationships should be equally fun and enjoyable for both people. If your friend or partner doesn't think your joking or teasing is funny—*it's not*. So before you start playing around, take a moment to consider your motives, as well as your partner or friend's state of mind and sense of humour.

Ask yourself the following questions:

- Do you feel calm, clear-headed, and connected to the other person?

- Is your true intent to communicate positive feelings—or are you taking a dig, expressing anger, or laughing at the other person's expense?
- Are you sure that the joke will be understood and appreciated?
- Are you aware of the emotional tone of the nonverbal messages you are sending? Are you giving off positive, warm signals or a negative, aggressive, or hostile tone?
- Are you sensitive to the nonverbal signals the other person is sending? Do they seem open and receptive to your humour, or closed-off and offended?
- Are you willing and able to back off if the other person responds negatively to the joke?
- If you say or do something that offends, is it easy for you to immediately apologize?

When conflict and disagreement throw a wrench in your relationships, humour and playfulness can help lighten things up and restore a sense of connection. Used skillfully and respectfully, playful humour can turn conflict into an opportunity for shared fun and intimacy. It allows you to get your point across without getting the other person's defenses up or hurting their feelings.

Humour and playfulness neutralize conflict by helping you:

- Interrupt the power struggle, instantly easing tension and allowing you to reconnect and regain perspective.
- Be more spontaneous. Shared laughter and play helps you break free from rigid ways of thinking and behaving, allowing you to see the problem in a new way and find a creative solution.
- Be less defensive. In playful settings, we hear things differently and can tolerate learning things about ourselves that we otherwise might find unpleasant or even painful.
- Let go of inhibitions. Laughter opens us up, freeing us to express what we truly feel and allowing our deep, genuine emotions to rise to the surface.

Humour and shared playfulness help you stay resilient in the face of life's challenges. But there are times when humour is *not* healthy—when it is used as a cover for avoiding, rather than coping with, painful emotions. Laughter can be a disguise for feelings of hurt, fear, anger, and disappointment that you don't want to feel or don't know how to express. You can be funny about the truth—but covering up the truth isn't funny. When you use humour and playfulness as a cover for other emotions, you create confusion and mistrust in your relationships.

For cues as to whether or not humour is being used to conceal other emotions, ask yourself the following questions:

- Do nonverbal communication signals—such as tone of voice, intensity, timing—feel genuinely humorous to you, or do you experience them as forced or "not right" somehow?
- Is humour the only emotion you routinely express, or is there a mixture of other emotions that at least occasionally includes sadness, fear, and anger?

Improving your playful communication skills
It's never too late to develop and embrace your playful, humorous side. Self-consciousness and concern for how you look and sound to others is probably a big factor that's limiting your playfulness. But as a baby, you were naturally playful; you didn't worry about the reactions of other people. You can reclaim your inborn playfulness by setting aside *regular, quality playtime*. The more you joke, play, and laugh—the easier it becomes.

Cultivating your sense of humour and playfulness
The process of learning to play depends on your preferences. Begin by observing what you already do that borders on fun or playful. For example:

- telling or listening to jokes
- watching funny movies or TV shows

- dancing around to music when you're alone
- singing in the shower
- daydreaming
- reading the funny pages

Then, you can try to incorporate more playful activities into your life. You could try taking an improvisation comedy class, throw a costume party, and even volunteer to provide the entertainment. The important thing is to find enjoyable activities that loosen you up and help you embrace your playful nature with other people.

Another excellent way to learn playfulness is to practice with the "experts" below:

- Play with animals. Puppies, kittens, and other animals—both young and old—are eager playmates and always ready to frolic. Play with a friends' pet, stop to play with a friendly animal in your neighbourhood, or consider getting a pet of your own.
- Play with customer service people. Most people in the service industry are social and you'll find that many will welcome playful banter.

As humour and play become an integrated part of your life, your creativity will flourish and new opportunities for playing with loved ones will occur to you daily.

*

Remember, keep your relationships fresh and exciting by joining in fun activities together, strengthening your emotional connection to yourself and each other.

Skill Five - The ability to resolve conflicts

The fifth skill for creating rewarding and lasting relationships is the ability to resolve conflicts in your relationships. The way you respond to differences and disagreements in personal and professional relationships can create hostility and irreparable rifts, or it can initiate the building of safety and trust. Your capacity to take conflict in your stride and to forgive easily is supported by your ability to manage stress, to be emotionally available, to communicate nonverbally, and to laugh easily.
Conflict in relationships can be a deal breaker and a heart breaker. Two people can't possibly always have the same needs, opinions and expectations—and that needn't be a bad thing! But when conflict is resolved in a healthy way, it can be a cornerstone for trust between people. When conflict isn't perceived as threatening or punishing, it fosters freedom, creativity, trust and safety in relationships.

Resolving conflict in a positive way involves:
- Staying focused in the present. When we are emotionally present and not holding on to old hurts and resentments, we can recognize the reality of a current situation and view it as a new opportunity for resolving old feelings about conflicts.
- Choosing your arguments. Consider what is worth arguing about and what is not. Pick your battles wisely.
- The ability to forgive. If you continue to be harmed protect yourself. But if not, conflict resolution involves suppressing the urge to punish.
- Ending conflicts that can't be resolved. It takes two people to keep an argument going. If you can't find common ground, let the argument go. Once you know how to remain emotionally present, and manage stress, you can avoid overreacting or under-reacting in emotionally charged situations. And with the aid of nonverbal communication and humour you

can catch and defuse many issues before they escalate into conflict, ie. agree to disagree.

Managing and Resolving Conflict

Conflict is a normal, and even healthy, part of relationships. After all, two people can't be expected to agree on everything at all times. Since relationship conflicts are inevitable, learning to deal with them in a healthy way is crucial. When conflict is mismanaged, it can harm the relationship. But when handled in a respectful and positive way, conflict provides an opportunity for growth, ultimately strengthening the bond between two people. By learning the skills you need for successful conflict resolution, you can keep your personal and professional relationships strong and growing.

Conflict arises from differences. It occurs whenever people disagree over their values, motivations, perceptions, ideas, or desires. Sometimes these differences look trivial. When a conflict triggers strong feelings, a deep personal and relational need is at the core of the problem, a need to feel safe and secure, a need to feel respected and valued, or a need for greater closeness and intimacy.

If you are out of touch with your own feelings or so stressed that you can only pay attention to a limited number of emotions, you won't be able to understand your own needs. If you don't understand your deep-seated needs, you will have a hard time communicating with others and staying in touch with what is really troubling you. For example, couples often argue about petty differences rather than what is really bothering them. In personal relationships, a lack of understanding about differing needs can result in distance, arguments, and break-ups. In workplace conflicts, differing needs are often at the heart of bitter disputes. When you can recognize the legitimacy of conflicting needs and become willing to examine them in an environment of compassionate understanding, it opens pathways to creative problem solving, team building, and improved relationships. When you resolve conflict and disagreement quickly and painlessly, mutual trust will flourish.

Successful conflict resolution depends on your ability to:

- Manage stress while remaining alert and calm. By staying calm, you can accurately read and interpret verbal and nonverbal communication.
- Control your emotions and behaviour. When you're in control of your emotions, you can communicate your needs without threatening, frightening, or punishing others.
- Pay attention to the feelings being expressed as well as the spoken words of others.
- Be aware of and respectful of differences. By avoiding disrespectful words and actions, you can resolve the problem faster.

Healthy and unhealthy ways of managing and resolving conflict

Conflict triggers strong emotions and can lead to hurt feelings, disappointment, and discomfort. When handled in an unhealthy manner, it can cause irreparable rifts, resentments, and break-ups.

Unhealthy responses to conflict are characterized by:

- An inability to recognize and respond to matters of great importance to the other person
- Explosive, angry, hurtful, and resentful reactions
- The withdrawal of love, resulting in rejection, isolation, shaming, and fear of abandonment
- The expectation of bad outcomes
- The fear and avoidance of conflict

But remember, when conflict is resolved in a healthy way, it increases our understanding of one another, builds trust, and strengthens our relationship bonds.

Healthy responses to conflict are characterized by:

- The capacity to recognize and respond to important matters
- A readiness to forgive and forget
- The ability to seek compromise and avoid retaliation
- A belief that resolution can support the interests and needs of both parties

Four key conflict resolution skills
The ability to successfully manage and resolve conflict depends on four key skills. Together, these four skills form a fifth skill that is greater than the sum of its parts: the ability to take conflict in stride and resolve differences in ways that build trust and confidence.

Conflict resolution skill 1: Quickly relieve stress
The capacity to remain relaxed and focused in tense situations is a vital aspect of conflict resolution. If you don't know how to stay centered and in control of yourself, you may become emotionally overwhelmed in challenging situations. Remember, the best way to rapidly and reliably relieve stress is through the senses: sight, sound, touch, taste, and smell. But each person responds differently to sensory input, so you need to find things that are soothing to you.

Conflict resolution skill 2: Recognize and manage your emotions.
Emotional awareness is the key to understanding yourself and others. If you don't know how you feel or why you feel that way, you won't be able to communicate effectively or smooth over disagreements. Although knowing your own feelings may seem simple, many people ignore or try to sedate strong emotions like anger, sadness, and fear. But your ability to handle conflict depends on being connected to these feelings. If you're afraid of strong emotions or if you insist on finding

solutions that are strictly rational, your ability to face and resolve differences will be impaired.

Conflict resolution skill 3: Improve your nonverbal communication skills
The most important information exchanged during conflicts and arguments is often communicated nonverbally. Nonverbal communication includes eye contact, facial expression, tone of voice, posture, touch, and gestures. When you're in the middle of a conflict, paying close attention to the other person's nonverbal signals may help you figure out what the other person is really saying. Respond in a way that builds trust, and get to the root of the problem. Simple nonverbal signals such as a calm tone of voice, a reassuring touch, or a concerned facial expression can go a long way toward defusing a heated exchange.

Conflict resolution skill 4: Use humour and play to deal with challenges
You can avoid many confrontations and resolve arguments and disagreements by communicating in a playful or humorous way. Humour can help you say things that might otherwise be difficult to express without creating another problem. However, it's important that you laugh *with* the other person, not *at* them. When humour and play is used to reduce tension and anger, reframe problems, and put the situation into perspective, the conflict can actually become an opportunity for greater connection and intimacy.

Tips for managing and resolving conflict
Managing and resolving conflict requires emotional maturity, self-control, and empathy. It can be tricky, frustrating, and even frightening. You can ensure that the process is as painless and positive as possible by sticking to the following conflict resolution guidelines:

• Make the relationship your priority. Maintaining and strengthening the relationship, rather than "winning" the argument, should always be your first priority. Be

52

respectful of the other person and his or her viewpoint.

- Focus on the present. If you're holding on to old hurts and resentments, your ability to see the reality of the current situation will be impaired. Rather than looking to the past and assigning blame, focus on what you can do in the here-and-now to solve the problem.
- Pick your battles. Conflicts can be draining, so it's important to consider whether the issue is really worthy of your time and energy. Maybe you don't want to surrender a parking space if you've been circling for fifteen minutes. But if there are dozens of spots, arguing over a single space is not worth it.
- Be willing to forgive. Resolving conflict is impossible if you're unwilling or unable to forgive.
- Know when to let something go. If you can't come to an agreement, agree to disagree. It takes two people to keep an argument going. If a conflict is going nowhere, you can choose to disengage and move on.

Ground rules
- Remain calm. Try not to overreact to difficult situations. By remaining calm it will be more likely that others will consider your viewpoint.

- Express feelings in words, not actions. Telling someone directly and honestly how you feel can be a very powerful form of communication. If you start to feel so angry or upset that you feel you may lose control, take a "time out" and do something to help yourself feel steadier.

- Be specific about what is bothering you. Vague complaints are hard to work on.

- Deal with only one issue at a time. Don't introduce other topics until each is fully discussed. This avoids the "kitchen sink" effect where people throw in all their complaints while not allowing anything to be resolved.

- No "hitting below the belt." Attacking areas of personal sensitivity creates an atmosphere of distrust, anger, and vulnerability.

- Avoid accusations. Accusations will cause others to defend themselves. Instead, talk about how someone's actions made you feel.

- Don't generalize. Avoid words like "never" or "always." Such generalizations are usually inaccurate and will heighten tensions.

- Avoid "make believe." Exaggerating or inventing a complaint - or your feelings about it - will prevent the real issues from surfacing. Stick with the facts and your honest feelings.

- Don't stockpile. Storing up lots of grievances and hurt feelings over time is counterproductive. It's almost impossible to deal with numerous old problems for which interpretations may differ. Try to deal with problems as they arise.

- Avoid clamming up. When one person becomes silent and stops responding to the other, frustration and anger can result. Positive results can only be attained with two-way communication.

Manage and resolve conflict by learning how to listen when people are upset. The words they use rarely convey the issues and needs at the heart of the problem. When we listen for what is felt as well as said, we connect more deeply to our own needs and emotions, and to those of other people. Listening in this way also strengthens us, informs us, and makes it easier for others to hear us.

Tips for being a better listener:

- Listen to the reasons the other person gives for being upset.

- Make sure you understand what the other person is telling you from his or her point of view.
- Repeat the other person's words, and ask if you have understood correctly.
- Ask if anything remains unspoken, giving the person time to think before answering.
- Resist the temptation to interject your own point of view until the other person has said everything he or she wants to say and feels that you have listened to and understood his or her message.

When listening to the other person's point of view, the following responses are often helpful:

- Encourage the other person to share his or her issues as fully as possible.
  "I want to understand what has upset you."
  "I want to know what you are really hoping for."
- Clarify the real issues, rather than making assumptions. Ask questions that allow you to gain this information, and which let the other person know you are trying to understand.
  "Can you say more about that?"
  "Is that the way it usually happens?"
- Re-state what you have heard, so you are both able to see what has been understood so far - it may be that the other person will then realize that additional information is needed.
  "It sounds like you weren't expecting that to happen."
- Reflect feelings - be as clear as possible.
  "I can imagine how upsetting that must have been."
- Validate the concerns of the other person, even if a solution is elusive at this time. Expressing appreciation can be a very powerful message if it is conveyed with integrity and respect.
  "I really appreciate that we are talking about this issue."
  "I am glad we are trying to figure this out."

*

Remember, building rewarding, lasting relationships is about staying calm and focused, regardless of the circumstances. It's about communicating clearly with the other person, understanding your motivations, feelings, needs and those of others. It's about being able to defuse arguments and repair wounded feelings and knowing how to add playfulness and joy in your relationships.

Together, the five skills of emotional intelligence help you build strong relationships, overcome challenges, and succeed at work and in life. The good news is that the skills of emotional intelligence can be learned by anyone, at anytime.